Issues in Medical Office Automation

George O. Obikoya

Abstract

Few physicians will doubt that information technology can potentially improve the operations of their practices and the quality of care they provide their patients. Progress in the development of clinical information systems has opened up even more avenues for physicians to improve their productivity, perform efficient operations, and increase their competitiveness and profitability. However, despite its benefits many physicians are yet to automate their practices. Indeed, the healthcare industry as a whole lags behind other information-intensive industries with regard to embracing information technology.

With physicians, various interest groups and the public increasingly averse to medical errors and patients keener to be more actively involved in their treatment, clinical information systems are likely to be increasingly utilized. Furthermore, the various issues stalling the widespread adoption of electronic medical records being resolved and cutting-edge technologies able to improve patient care developed.

For physicians to use computer systems more and be able to make informed choices regarding which to acquire in order to improve their medical practices, they need to be aware of the evolution of new computer solutions, and the many salient technical, clinical, and other issues currently relevant to computerizing the medical office. This paper explores some of these issues, discusses recent advances in relevant IT, and suggests ways to improving current medical office automation practices.

Issues in medical office automation

Introduction

Innovations in information technology (IT) are creating new opportunities for physicians

to meet the demands of contemporary medical practice.[1] Salient technical, financial,

management and other issues are emerging in tandem with the evolution of computer systems.

Some of these issues are government regulations that bear directly on medical practice. Others

are changing public attitudes that will likely impact elements of current practice. Yet others

reveal technology trends required for high a quality, competitive practice. Physicians also need

to be cognizant of these issues and of the need to be able to make informed choices regarding

which computer systems to acquire in order to improve their medical practices.[2]

Advances in IT

Significant clinical and economic benefits accrue from implementing "virtual radiology,"

in which traditional film-based operations do not use films and a central commercial Picture

archival and communication system (PACS) is integrated with a practice's information and

transcription systems[3]. Dictation is redundant with voice recognition systems implemented[1].

Automation generates value added services for the patients as well as economic benefits for the

practice[4]. It enhances productivity, improves quality of care, and reduces operational costs and

administrative overhead [5, 6] Paperwork can be minimized and patient, financial and
administrative information better managed with cutting-edge database management

solutions.[7]Billing, scheduling, and insurance reporting operations can be streamlined,

customized, and more efficiently run[8]

Enterprise resource planning solutions (ERP), web-enabled, outsourced, or hosted by an application service provider (ASP) can integrate and facilitate the control of a practice's units and functions[9]. Enterprise intranet solutions and the Internet can be integrated enabling physically dispersed healthcare entities to share information that is also accessible on demand at points of care.[10] Due to their wide application, ERP software systems have an extensive software base and can be very costly to implement. Cheaper systems can now be obtained and several ERP Systems such as Compiere and SQL Ledger are available for free as Open Source systems under a royalty-free license and can be customized to suit the practice's needs.

Advances in wireless and mobile computing technologies and their applications and increased computer power and speed are significantly impacting health care communications.[11] Web technology solutions enable physician practice to collect patient information and transfer it to hospital applications for specialized investigation and other purposes without creating a tedious paper trail. This facilitates pre-certification, advanced beneficiary notices, and confirmation of payer eligibility, and prevents service denials and delays. Advances in broadband access technology such as greater bandwidth, improved quality of service capabilities, multicast, and applications availability enable physicians gain speedy access to vital information. They also have a variety of choices of broadband access technologies, including Digital Subscriber Lines (DSL), Cable, wireless, and lately Ethernet or Fiber. Artificial Intelligence techniques such as expert systems, [12] artificial neural networks (ANN), [13] and data mining [14] are enhancing physicians' productivity and improving the quality of patient care. Physicians also use a variety of ergonomically sophisticated handheld devices and software to facilitate their work[15]. Bluetooth, a high-speed, low-power microwave wireless link technology, designed to easily connect phones, laptops, personal digital assistants (PDA) and other portable equipments improves efficiency as physicians can access and store information, print documents, and perform other functions while away from their computers without the need to connect cables to peripherals. Telemedicine is enabling remote monitoring of patients' blood pressure, blood sugar, renal dialysis, and asthma. Hailey et al highlighted its clinical and economic advantages in their systematic review of 66 studies of the benefits of telemedicine applications.[16] Computer telephony that enables the electronic transmission of voice, fax, or other information facilitates patient contact, reduces operating costs, and enhances staff efficiency and productivity. Automation frees-up clerical staff to assist with in-office patients and relieves physicians of mundane tasks, enabling them to better focus on patient care.

Despite its clear benefits, many physicians have not yet automated their practices. Indeed, the healthcare industry as a whole lags behind other industries in adopting IT, according to some estimates by at least a decade[17]. A recent study of IT sophistication among Canadian medical centers showed functional sophistication to be of high-moderate levels, technological sophistication of low levels, and integration sophistication even lower levels[18]. There are several reasons for the apparent lack of interest in IT by medical professionals, including, reluctance to jettison hand-written prescribing and other entrenched practices, technophobia, uncertainties over whether or not automation creates value and how to proceed with it. Physicians are also generally unfamiliar with the operations of vendors and the software market. Other issues include costs, privacy, legal and ethical, safety, training, maintenance, and the apparent inflexibility of earlier office software programs[19]. While these are pertinent issues, embracing IT creates significant opportunities for medical practices to be more competitive, to provide high quality patient care, and to increase the bottom line. Medicare's 1990 policy to pay claims submitted electronically before paper-based claims spurred physicians' interests in practice management systems (PMS), designed to assist physicians track patient demographic, payment and insurance information, although the adoption of later applications such as electronic medical records (EMR), document management solutions, electronic dictations, and laboratory solutions has been much slower.

Medical practices are under more pressure to raise customer service levels while simultaneously attempting to control or cut costs. Physicians need to be more acquainted with basic practice software architecture, implementation, and maintenance. They need to be able to justify the costs they are about to incur by calculating the current cost of the tasks to be automated then estimating the cost of the tasks under the proposed system. They also need to be able to evaluate software, hence be able to drive the market to develop packages that conform to their needs and minimal quality criteria.[20]

Planning

The need for broad-based systematic planning and control procedures such as systems life cycles becomes more acute as medical office automation activities become more complex and interrelated. Proper planning before IT investment will undeniably help prevent wastage of scarce financial resources. Physicians should first determine the operations that need automation. For examples, office visit, billing, appointments, laboratory and therapy scheduling, electronic medical record (EMR) management, insurance reimbursements, and prescription tracking can all but need not all be automated. They should also know the software and hardware needed and their costs, how good the current system performs, training and maintenance costs, and the costs of integrating the legacy and new systems. IT can no doubt provide the essential tools to run a modern practice but the physician needs a clear vision of what the practice should be now and years down the road. The blueprint of the practice's IT architecture, which establishes its technical computing, information management, and networking platform, should show not only the IT design but how its various components coalesce. The IT architecture determines the practice's spectrum of IT and its business options.

Planning for a new system or for upgrading an existing one requires addressing three main elements of IT architecture. These elements are the processing systems architecture, which defines the technical standards for the hardware, operating systems, and applications software required; the network architecture, which defines the links between the practice's communications units for information flow internally and between its entities and; the data architecture, which defines data organization for storage, retrieval, and accessibility. Together these elements form the basis for integrating the practice's IT resources. Physicians might however, ultimately adopt any of traditional approaches such as batch, transactional or messaging technology or newer ones such as service-oriented architecture (SOA) or zero-latency enterprise technology.

An effective architecture allows as much vendor-independence as practicable and is capable of rationalizing the confusion of multiple vendors and incompatible technologies, and incorporates current and imminent industry standards. Rather than architecture-centered planning, however, physicians can choose the technology base best suited to a specific application based on cost, efficiency, speed, and ease of use. This is a reasonable move provided integrating the applications for data or network resource-sharing purposes is not required.

Implementation

The technical details involved in defining and implementing a practice's IT solutions can be daunting due to a variety of reasons such as systems' incompatibilities, lack of consensus over standards, and the multiplicity of vendor-unique applications and services and of vendors.

However, developments in standards such as the agreement between IBM and its competitors on compatibility with important IBM architectures and vendor-free standards particularly OSI and UNIX have eased matters. Selecting a common set of tools for personal computers, including the operating system and a "suite" of applications to facilitate reliance on fewer standards linking these applications, can define, and implement architecture.

Service-oriented architectures (SOA) and event-driven designs are more commonly used and will likely rely more for their interfaces on Web services standards such as Web Services Description Language (WSDL) or Simple Object Access Protocol (SOAP) as they evolve and mature. New software products, enterprise service buses (ESB), which support but do not require web services, are able to resolve the technical difficulties hindering the interoperability of web server and application server platforms caused by incompatibilities and deficient official standards. Large physician and group practices should consider using an ESB as a middleware backbone particularly when their SOA applications will comprise more than two different application servers. They should also consider the same approach when asynchronous communication will be used and when an application set will encompass a mix of Web services and other forms of inter-program communications.[21] To make costs more manageable, physicians can implement solutions in incremental phases starting with basic IT infrastructure and low-level front-office applications before implementing increasingly advanced clinical-oriented and EMR applications.

Workflow management

Workflow management can create value for medical practices. The more complex a workflow, and the more physically dispersed its units, the more benefit will likely accrue from automation. Workflow automation can reduce lag time, minimize errors, assure best practices, and in some cases provide an audit trail. More sophisticated front-and back-office practice management solutions continue to be made available through Application Service Providers (ASPs), a variety of software, thin-client and web-deployed systems. Physicians need to define the workflow processes they want to manage and their current problems, for examples excessive paperwork, burdensome file storage and retrieval systems, message follow-up pile-ups, and delayed request refills. They must then choose an appropriate and cost-effective workflow management system capable of streamlining their practices' overall operations and of enhancing productivity, cutting costs and improving the quality patient care.[22] Importantly, the new system should be adapted to suite the practices' strategic and tactical objectives rather than vice versa. For example, if often unable to respond promptly to phone calls, emails, and other messages that might require urgent patient-related attention, physicians can use a workflow system capable of recognizing and prioritizing messages that demand the physician's immediate attention and those other staff can handle.

Electronic Medical Records (EMR)

EMR is crucial to workflow management. It integrates patients' demographic, insurance and clinical information and enables multiple and timely access to these resources including at

the point of care. EMR has yet to be implemented in many practices [23] despite its proven validity for use in general practice [24] its many clinical benefits,[25]and the increasing favorable public attitude towards its use. [26] Confusion over the large number of choices and fear that mistakes may prove costly and frustrating are some of the reasons reportedly hindering EMR adoption.[27] Other notable concerns include cost, hardware and software failures, conversion hardships, confidentiality and liability issues, training needs, and physicians' attitudes[29].

Efforts to address the issues stalling the widespread adoption of EMR continue. Privacy is protected by statutes in the U.S and most of the western world [30, 31, 32] The slowness of physicians

to accept EMR[33] and the deficient coding and hierarchic structure of existing medical vocabulary

also hinder its widespread use[34]. The use of the digital ink in telephone messaging and for

consultation might be one way to facilitate EMR acceptance by physicians[35]. So will focus on the
interface solutions, some of which are currently available in the form of standards: IP, HL7 /

ASTM, DICOM, LOINC, SNOMED, although are yet to be fully embraced.[36]

CPOE and patient safety

Up to 98,000 preventable deaths per year occur in the U.S due to medical errors[37]. Over

30% of hand-written prescriptions had errors that required correction by a pharmacist[38]. The use

of computerized physician order entry (CPOE) reduces medical errors[39]. Most mistakes occur in

the least computerized part of the prescribing process, physician order entry[40]. With a minimal
learning curve, physicians using CPOE enter orders into a computerized system whence it can be

processed by other applications to ensure dosages are correct, there are no allergies or other

contraindications to the use of the medications, even calculate a patient-specific dose, the

optimum dose for the patient's age, sex, weight and other medical factors. CPOE reduced errors

by 55%, from 10.7 to 4.9 per 1,000 patient days and rates of serious medication errors fell by

88% at Harvard's Brigham and Women's Hospital.[39]

Despite their benefits, CPOE use is yet to be widespread. CPOE is not cheap to

implement and may be out of reach of small practices but their return on investment more than

justifies the cost.[40] CPOE implementation cost $1.9 million with annual maintenance expenses of

$500,000 at the 735-bed Brigham and Women's Hospital. However, it saved about $500,000 and

between $5 million to $10 million per year in direct and indirect costs, respectively[39]. The public

is increasingly concerned about medical errors [41] as are some powerful interest groups.[42] CPOE is currently used by less than 5 percent of hospitals, its use estimated to rise in the next five years

to 12 percent[42].

Leading healthcare and consumer organizations have endorsed 30 specific practices that

healthcare organizations should implement in order to improve patient safety. They include

adopting CPOE and encouraging pharmacists to be more actively involved in the medication-use

process, including interpretation and review of medical orders and administration or monitoring

of medications.[43]

Standards

Both vendors and users are increasingly acknowledging the need for a comprehensive set

of vendor-free standards. The Open Systems Interconnection model, or OSI, is an abstract

reference model and a standards effort for transmitting messages between two end-users in a

telecommunication network. It aims to facilitate communication between hardware and software

systems despite differences in underlying architectures. It is the internationally recognized

framework for developing networking standards such as the Specification and description

language (SDL). SDL is the premier language for real time systems development.[44] Standards

evolve with technologies hence will likely be different for legacy and new systems. This should

be borne in mind in defining the IT architecture in order to safeguard current investments and to

ensure that new ones are value-added. Because technology evolves much faster than the

standards, ensuring that the architecture does not hinder the practice's growth or the

implementation of a novel solution could pose a dilemma.

The U.S. Department of Health and Human Services (HHS) has mandated the Institute of

Medicine to design a standardized model of an electronic healthcare record (EHR). Health Level

Seven Inc., a standards development organization will evaluate the model[45], which will be

available in 2004 and distributed free to all entities of the U.S. healthcare system. HHS has also

signed a $32 million five-year contract with the College of American Pathologists (CAP) to

license its 340,000 concept-strong standardized medical vocabulary system, SNOMED

(Systematized Nomenclature of Medicine). The National Library of Medicine will administer the

agreement, which should encourage more practitioners to embrace EMR, and provide a database

of standardized medical and clinical terminology and a common communication platform. The

XML standards facilitates cross-enterprise communication between applications, more integrated

ERP and customized solutions.[46]

Costs and the revenue cycle

Medical office automation is becoming increasingly versatile and more affordable and

cost-effective.[47] New York's Memorial Sloan-Kettering Cancer Center saved $365,000 in

physical space, microfilm, and media costs the first year it implemented electronic remittance

posting and imaging in patient accounting. It later added EDI to manage claim-status

information, thereby enhancing client service and its patients accounting operations.[48] Billing

errors, insurance underpayments, denials and self-pay bad debt cost hospitals about 13 percent in

lost revenue annually[49]. Physicians can reduce costs and improve operational efficiency by

automating manual financial and clinical processes[50]. The rising cost of healthcare delivery is due

in part to problems with the revenue cycle. [51] The cycle starts the moment a physician sees a
patient in his/her practice, goes well past the patient's discharge, and persists until the analysis of

the success or failure ratios of claims by each individual payer. Archaic data collection and

management systems, laborious manual and paper-based claims rework, appeals, and account

follow-up adversely affect the revenue cycle and compromise profitability.[52]

Inefficient front-end processes cause many claims rejections, at least 90% of which can be prevented by collecting accurate patient information using web-based, work-list queue management, and HIPAA compliance in the U.S. Other appropriate solutions are those capable of efficient claims generation and processing and of verifying eligibility and checking credit ratings and addresses upfront.[53] Practices can build their own data with an automated claims system. They can also identify and correct errors before claims submission, minimizing rejections and facilitating reimbursements with an automated claims system. Revenue cycle technology enhances financial success and patient satisfaction.[54]

The Patient Friendly Billing Project underscores the need for improving patient satisfaction using appropriate automation. The Healthcare Financial Management Association and the American Hospital Association started the project in 2002. Its goals include providing clean, concise and correct information to healthcare consumers.[55] The Summer2003 Report of the project gave 14 recommendations to healthcare providers to create a more patient-focused billing and collection process including instituting customer service standards, informing patients in advance regarding their financial obligations; consolidating bills where possible; and creating online billing and payment portals.

Physicians also need to monitor and ensure receipt of expected payments from insurance firms particularly as third-party denials are common and often expensive. Contract management systems can automate this task improving workflow and enabling physicians to amend and update contract rules. It is important for the system to have denial analysis and reporting capabilities to monitor payer performance. It should also allow retrospective monitoring of denial frequency and type from insurers to minimize denial volume and to enhance decision-making and productivity. Automation must result in enough reduction in variable costs to justify the fixed costs of implementation. Software change alone is unlikely to achieve revenue cycle goals. Meeting staff, knowledge, and process re-engineering requirements will maximize the benefits of software acquisitions.[56]

Vendors

Software vendors are not difficult to find as surfing the Internet will show. The problem is finding one that will deliver fully functional, reliable and scalable software. One also backed by competent technical support, sold at reasonable prices, and that meet return on investments (ROI) and total cost of ownership (TOC) expectations. Besides searching the Internet, which is likely to produce vendor sites with the vendor's sales information, other helpful sources for finding vendors include personal contacts, computer consultants, industry trade groups and selection services. Personal contacts might want to genuinely help but have antiquated data about the vendors. Computer consultants can be involved in the entire or parts of software development and/or acquisition process and are likely to be current and to know the industry well. Data from trade groups will likely be unbiased but might be outdated. Selection services tend to have current knowledge bases of process features and vendor attributes and most likely to best match the practice's requirements with vendors' capabilities. However, their services tend to be expensive. The source of vendor information not withstanding, a Request for Proposal (RFP) should be part of any contract signed with the vendor.

Existing proprietary software are often comprehensive vertical market management software. Vertical market software is software designed to service the specific needs of an industry. Typically, it bundles all of, for example, a medical practice's application needs into one comprehensive package. Vertical market applications often target smaller firms and practices. There may be problems with these applications integrating well with others. The software market is undergoing structural changes that will result in notable changes in software vendors'

licensing and sales practices in the long haul. Software is becoming less construed as a physical

package with strictly specified attributes and functions and more as a service. This is due to a

variety of reasons, including firms acquiring software based on average and actual rather than

peak usage patterns thereby cutting costs and the exponential growth of the Internet opening

avenues for expanded applications deployment.[57]

As software vendors move away from the conventional software licensing policies such

as licensing software use based on the number of physical PC's or workstations within a firm

towards more flexible licensing terms to meet their clients' the usage needs, physicians need to

be able to estimate their needs in order to rationalize purchase. Network licensing is in on the

rise, which means that a hospital's entities can share licenses and acquire software as per

concurrent usage. Concurrent based licensing is, however, not suited to all applications,

particularly mission critical applications such as those used in hospitals that denying access to

could lead to catastrophic consequences. Further, because usage pattern may be unknown makes

it difficult to determine the appropriate licensing mix. Some vendors prefer a usage-based or

pay-per-use licensing model, which by purchasing licenses based on actual usage prevents denial

of service and increases account penetration. You can purchase overdraft licenses to supplement

the main license.[57]

Maintenance and technical support

Proprietary vertical market software may or may not provide source code to customers,

although often does with highly customized applications built for large clients, albeit often

hinged on restrictive non-disclosure agreements. Such agreements practically and legally make

the vendor alone available to support the product. Under these circumstances, the physician can forget about software support, pay the vendor's maintenance fees for even inferior services, or shop around for new vendors. This is why some physicians opt for open source software. Anyone who program in the language can maintain the software.[58]

Evaluation

Vital to any practice's success is the ability to obtain useful information and feedback about its performance.[59] In particular, physicians need to start to appreciate that non-value-adding work activities compromise their bottom lines. The need to provide data and reports throughout the continuum of care cannot be overemphasized. These resources capture on-going operations and facilitate re-engineering and forward planning. Physicians must align the IT and control systems of their practices with planning and decision-making.[60]

A major problem with measuring the information management & technology (IM&T) function is that infrastructure investments cannot be cost justified on a return on investment (ROI) basis. A viable alternative is the balanced scorecard (BSC), a method of evaluating corporate performance from the financial, internal business process, customer, and the learning and growth perspectives[61]. The Joint Commission on Accreditation of Healthcare Organizations mandates accredited organizations to use a performance measurement system, the ORYX initiative, for both internal performance control and benchmarking against external performance.[62] Regular performance appraisals help practices maintain standards and achieve their overall goals. Members of the American Academy of Family Physicians (AAFP) now have Web access to national data that enables them to benchmark their practice's performance against similar practices of similar size, payer types and patient mix, and to recognize over- and under-coding instances as well as identify opportunities for generate more revenue.[63]

Conclusion

IT tailored to the individual needs of medical practices improves the quality of medical care delivery. New pricing models such as utility computing, software as a service, and on-demand computing, can significantly lessen IT investments costs. Computer-based access to patients' full drug profiles and alerts about likely prescribing problems reduces the rate of

initiating probable improper prescriptions.[64] Computerized decision-making support can also minimize drug-related adverse events [65] and make drug selection more cost-effective[66]. Cost, privacy, time, legal liability, and training are some of the main concerns of practitioners about office automation. However, the medical community can no longer afford to ignore the benefits of the computerized practice. Doctors and the public at large are increasingly concerned about

medical errors.[67] Patients now demand the enforcement of error-prevention practices such as the use of bar codes and are keener to be active participants in their management.[68] These developments will likely increase the implementation of medical office automation in the near future.

References

1. Dowdle, J, (2002) The computer in office medical practice, *Clin Sports Med,* Apr. 21:231-5.

2. Tucker, G (2002) What works: all-round efficiency, Massachusetts OB/GYN practice improves its financial and administrative health with practice management software, *Health Manag Technol* 2003 May 24: 44-6.

3. Siegal, SL. Reiner, BI (2003) Filmless radiology at the Baltimore VA Medical Center: a 9-year retrospective, *Computerized Medical Imaging and Graphics*, 27: (2-3), March-June 2003, Pages 101-109

4. Sinaiko, J (2002) Improve compliance and financial performance at the same time, *J Med Pract Manage* 2002 Nov-Dec 18:3 155-8

5. Dunn, R (2001), When health information and fiscal management meet, *J AHIMA* 2001 Jan 72:1 37-41

6. McCarthy, EL (2002) Physician office productivity improvement through operations analysis and process redesign, *J Ambul Care Manage* 2002 Oct 25:4 37-52

7. Silver, D. (2002) Doing away with paper. Part 1--Advice for setting up fully computerized medical records, *Aust Fam Physician* 2002 Jun 31: 521-6

8. Guyton, E.M., Lund, C. (2003) Transforming the revenue cycle, *Healthc Financ Manage* 2003 Mar 57:3 72-8

9. Jenkins E.K, Christenson E (2001) ERP (enterprise resource planning) systems can streamline healthcare business functions. *Healthc Financ Manage* 2001 May 55:5 48-52

10. Baldwin, G. (2000) How the Internet is changing practice management systems, *Health Data Manag* 2000 Oct 8:10 42-4, 48-50, 52

11. McClay, J (2003) Wireless computing and health care *J Med Pract Manage* 2003 Mar-Apr 18:5 250-5

12. Thornett A.M. Computer decision support systems in general practice. *International Journal of Information Management,* February 2001: 21(1); 39-47

13. Lisboa, P.J.G., (2002), A review of evidence of health benefit from artificial neural networks in medical intervention *Neural Networks,* 2002, 15:1:11-39

14. Kiel, J.M., (2000) Data mining and modeling: power tools for physician practices, *MD Comput* 2000 May-Jun 17:3 33-4

15. Adatia, F. Bedard, P.L., (2003) 'Palm reading '2. Hand-held software for physicians, *CMAJ* 2003 Mar 168: 727-34

16. Hailey D., Roine R, Ohinmaa A (2002) Systematic review of evidence for the benefits of telemedicine, *J Telemed Telecare* 2002 8 Suppl 1: 1-30

17. Raghupathi W. Health Care Information Systems – Introduction, *CACM,* August 1997; 40 (8): 80-82.

18. Pare, G. Sicotte, C (2002) Information technology sophistication in health care: an instrument validation study among Canadian hospitals, *International Journal of Medical Informatics,* 63: (3) October 2001, Pp. 205-223

19. Ashcroft, R, (2001) Ethical, Legal and Social Issues facing the West London Database Project: A Review of the Literature, NHS Executive London Regional Office 2001

20. Englin, I. (2002) Model of data structure and flow in general practice: a guide to evaluation of practice management software. *Aus J Rural Health* 2000 Feb 8: 29-34

21. Gartner's Application Integration and Middleware Strategies Research Note DF-18-7304, 9 December 2002, Available at: http://www.gartner.com/gc/webletter/sonic/issue1/article1.html Accessed on: August 13, 2003

22. Spath, P. (2002) Use system analysis for lasting improvements, *Hosp Case Manag* 2002 Oct 10:150, 159-60

23. Dansky, K.H., Gamm, L.D., Barsukiewicz, C.K. (1999) Electronic medical records: are physicians ready? *J Healthc Manag* 1999 Nov-Dec 44:440-54; discussion 454-5

24. Hassey, A., Gerrett, D., Wilson, A., (2001) A survey of validity and utility of electronic patient records in a general practice, *BMJ* 2001 June 9; 322 (7299): 1401–1405

25. Lazarus R, Kleinman KP, Dashevsky I, et. al (2001), Using automated medical records for rapid identification of illness syndromes (syndromic surveillance): the example of lower respiratory infection. *BMC Public Health,* 2001;1(1): 9

26. Martin, Shelley, Canadians don't appear to fear electronic medical records. *CMAJ,* 2001 June 12; 164 (12): 1739

27. Silver, D. (2002) Doing away with paper. Part 1-Advice for setting up fully computerized medical records, *Aust Fam Physician* 2002 Jun 31:521-6

28. Mushan, C., Omstein, SM., Jenkins, RG., (1995) Family practice educators' perceptions of computer-based patient records *Fam Med* 1995 Oct 27:571-5

29. Medical Records Institute: Fifth annual Survey of EHR Trends and Usage, Available at: www.rsleads.com/308ht-225, Accessed on September10, 2003.

30. General Overview of standards for privacy of individually identifiable health information OCR HIPAA Privacy December 2002, Revised April 3, 2003. Available at: http://www.hhs.gov/ocr/hipaa/guidelines/overview.pdf, Accessed on August 10, 2003

31. Health Canada: Toward Electronic Health Records Office of Health and the *Information Highway Health Canada January 2001*

32. HMSO (1998) Data Protection Act 1998, Chapter 29, Available at: http://www.hmso.gov.uk/acts/acts1998/19980029.htm, Accessed on: August 10, 2003

33. Hertzberg, J (2000) Computerized patient records: current and future opportunities. *J Med Pract Manage* 2000 Mar-Apr 15:250-5

34. Chute, C.G. Cohn, S.P., and Campbell, J.R. (1998) A Framework for Comprehensive Health Terminology Systems in the United States: Development Guidelines, Criteria for Selection, and Public Policy Implications. *J Am Med Inform Assoc.* 1998 November; 5 (6): 503–510

35. Arvary, G.J., (1999) The Limited Use of Digital Ink in the Private-sector Primary Care Physician's Office, *J Am Med Inform Assoc.* 1999 Mar; 6(2): 134-142.

36. McDonald, C.J.,(1997)The Barriers to Electronic Medical Record Systems and How to Overcome Them. *J Am Med Inform Assoc,* 1997 May; 4 (3): 213–221

37. Institute of Medicine To Err Is Human: Building a Safer Health System. Washington, DC: National Academy Press; 2000.

38. Bates DW, Cullen DJ, Laird N, et al. Incidence of adverse drug events and potential adverse drug events: implications for prevention, *JAMA,* 1995; 274: 29-34

39. Bates DW, Teich JM, Lee J, Seger D, Kuperman GJ, Ma Luf N, Boyle D, Leape, The impact of computerized physician order entry on medication error prevention *JAMA* 1999; 6: 313-21

40. Hultman, J.A., Baum, N., (2000) Practice automation and medical errors *Cost Qual* Sep 6:3 21-3

41. Classen, D (2000) Patient safety, thy name is quality *Trustee* 2000 Oct 53:12-5, 1

42. Birkmeyer, JD, Birkmeyer CM, Wennberg, DE, Young MP, Leapfrog safety standards: potential benefits of universal adoption. The Leapfrog Group, Washington, DC: 2000.

43. Safe Practices for Better Healthcare: A Consensus Report from the National Quality Forum (NQF) (2003), Available at: www.rsleads.com/308ht-223 , Accessed on September 10, 2003.

44. Reed, R. (2001) Notes on SDL-2000 for the new millennium, *Computer Networks*, 35(6)May 2001, Pages 709-720

45. General Overview of standards for privacy of individually identifiable health information OCR HIPAA Privacy December 2002, Revised April 3, 2003. Available at: http://www.hhs.gov/ocr/hipaa/guidelines/overview.pdf, Accessed on September16, 2003

46. Stead, W.W., Miller, R.A., Musen, M.A., Hersh, W.R., (2000) Integration and Beyond Linking Information from Disparate Sources and into Workflow, *J Am Med Inform Assoc.* 2000 Mar; 7(2): 135-145.

47. Lowes, R (2003) Build an EMR for next to nothing. *Med Econ* Jun 6 80:11 29-30.

48. McBride J.S., Moynihan J.J. (1999) EDI and imaging automate the business office. *Healthc Financ Manage* 1999 Jan 53:62-4

49. Jaklevic M.C., (2001) Revenue stopper. Bungled billing system conversions are plaguing the hospital industry. *Mod Healthc* 2001 Jul 2 31:27 36-8

50. Fee, DN,(2002) Success with APCs. *Healthc Financ Manage* 2002 Sep 56:68-72

51. Runy, LA (2003) Revenue cycle management *Hosp Health Netw* 2003 Jun 77:51-6

52. Eden, K.B., (2002), Selecting IT for physicians' practices: A cross-sectional study, *BMC Med Inform Decis Mak.* 2002; 2(1): 4.

53. Bose, R. (2003) Knowledge management-enabled health care management systems: capabilities, infrastructure, and decision-support *Expert Systems with Applications* 24(1); Jan. 2003, Pages 59-71

54. Cox, M (2003) Money multiplies. Revenue cycle solutions lead three-tiered update of healthcare

system's business office. *Health Manag Technol* 2003 Jan 24:58, 61

55. The Patient Friendly Billing Project, Available at: http://www.patientfriendlybilling.org/, Accessed on September16, 2003

56. Eden, K.B. (2002) Selecting information technology for physicians' practices: a cross-sectional study, *BMC Med Inform Decis Mak,* 2002; 2(1): 4.

57. Kiel, J.M. (200) Buy software or "pay-per-view": the ASP option. *MD Comput* 2000 Jul-Aug 17:4 27-8

58. Mads, W.M. Affordable biocomputing for everyone: using the Internet, freeware and open-source software *Trends in Biochemical Sciences,* 2002, 27:11:586-588

59. Malayeff, J., Kaminsky, F.C., Jubinville, A., Fen, CA (2002) A guide to using performance measurement systems for continuous improvement, *J Healthc Qual* 2001 Jul-Aug 23:4 33-7

60. Michelman, J.E., Rausch, P.E., Barton, T.L. (1999) Value measurement in health care: a new perspective *Healthc Financ Manage* 1999 Aug 53:48-53

61. Protti, D (2002) A proposal to use a balanced scorecard to evaluate Information for Health: an information strategy for the modern NHS (1998–2005) *Computers in Biology and Medicine,* 32: (3) May 2002, Pages 221-236)

62. Hanold, L.S., Koss, R.G., Loeb, J.M. (2000) The ORYX initiative: goals and potential application to physician quality-improvement efforts, *Tex Med* 2000 Oct 96:84-7

63. American Academy of Family Physicians (AAFP), Available at Physcape's Web site at www.aafp.org/x21844.xml, Accessed on August 11, 2003

64. Tamblyn R, Huang A, Perreault R, Jacques A, Roy D, Hanley J, McLeod P, Laprise R (2003) The medical office of the 21st century (MOXXI): effectiveness of computerized decision-making support in reducing inappropriate prescribing in primary care *CMAJ.* 2003 Sep 16;169

(6):549-556.

65. Raschke RA, Gollihare B, Wunderlich TA, Guidry JR, Leibowitz AI, Peirce JC, et al. A computer alert system to prevent injury from adverse drug events: Development and evaluation in a community teaching hospital, *JAMA* 1998; 280:1317-20

66. Evans RS, Pestotnik SL, Classen DC, Clemmer TP, Weaver LK, Orme JF, et al. A computer-assisted management program for antibiotics and other anti-infective agents. *N Engl J Med* 1998; 338:232-8.

67. Blendon R.J, DesRoches, C.M., Brodie, M., Benson, J.M., Rosen, A.B., Schneider, E., Altman, D.E., Zapert, K., Hermann, M.J., Steffenson, A.E. (2002) Views of practicing physicians and the public on medical errors. *N Engl J Med* 2002 Dec 12 347:24 1933-40

68. Barry MJ. Involving patients in medical decisions: how can physicians do better? *JAMA* 1999; 282: 23567.